WALKING
IN
HIGH
VIBRATION

TITO JUNIOR BANCE

Published and Manufactured by Softwood Books
EU Responsible person: Maddy Glenn
Office 2, Wharfside House, Prentice Road, Stowmarket, Suffolk,
IP14 1RD
www.softwoodbooks.com
hello@softwoodbooks.com

EU Rep:
Authorised Rep Compliance Ltd., Ground Floor, 71 Lower Baggot
Street, Dublin, D02 P593, Ireland
www.arccompliance.com
info@arccompliance.com

Paperback ISBN: 978-1-0369-2498-0

Dedicated to Sarina

For my daughter,
whose light reminds me daily of the beauty in simply being.
May you always know your worth, walk in your truth,
and trust the wisdom within your soul.

You are my greatest teacher and my most sacred gift.
This book is a prayer for your freedom, your joy, and your highest
vibration.

With all my love,
Daddy

Contents

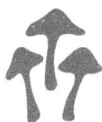

INTRODUCTION:

A Call to Remember

You didn't find this book by accident.

Something led you here — a feeling, a question, a longing. Maybe it was a moment of stillness. Maybe it was heartbreak. Maybe it was simply the quiet voice inside whispering, "there's more than this".

This book is not here to teach you who to become.

It's here to remind you who you already are.

You are light. You are energy. You are spirit walking through the human experience. And somewhere deep within you, you already know that.

We live in a world that pulls us away from that truth. We're taught to chase success, to fear stillness, to forget our divinity. But your soul never forgets. That's why you feel the call to something higher. That's why you're here.

Walking in High Vibrations is not just a book — it's a journey. A spiritual roadmap back to your truth. Back to peace. Back to presence. Back to the flow of the universe.

You'll explore the energy body, the subconscious mind, the art of letting go, the magic of manifestation, the wisdom in your wounds, and the power of faith. You'll learn not only how to raise your vibration but how to live in it, move with it, and become a living light for others.

Take what resonates. Leave the rest. Let this be a gentle guide, not a strict rulebook. Let your soul lead the way.

This isn't about becoming someone new.

It's about remembering the divine being you've always been.

You're not just walking through life.

You're walking in high vibrations.

Welcome home.

CHAPTER 1:

The Call to Stillness

There comes a point in life where the noise of the world just becomes too loud. The pressures, expectations, stress, and distractions start to drown out the whisper of your soul. That whisper, soft and subtle, is the call to stillness. It's the moment when the soul nudges you to pause, to reflect, and to remember who you truly are.

This call doesn't always show up gently; it can come through heartbreak, through burnout, through grief, or a quiet sadness that you can't explain. It may come after you've achieved everything you thought you wanted and still feel an emptiness inside. It's the universe reminding you that it's time to go within.

Stillness is where you find yourself again.

We live in a world that thrives on speed. We're always moving, always doing, always trying to prove something. But healing doesn't happen in the noise. Awakening doesn't come when you're scrolling, rushing, and constantly distracted. It comes in the silence. In the breath. In the now.

Meditation is not about becoming something new, it's about remembering who you already are beneath the thoughts, the worries, the roles you play. It's coming back home to the Self.

In stillness, you discover that you are more than your name, more than your job, more than your past. You are energy. You are light. You are consciousness. You are connected to all things and everything is connected to you.

Why We Meditate

Meditation is the doorway. Through it, we can begin to heal, grow, release, and reconnect. It is the most powerful tool we have to raise our vibration, to awaken the spirit, and to clear the fog from the mind. It's not about forcing the mind to go quiet. It's about letting go and allowing yourself to just be.

You can meditate to:

- Heal old wounds, emotionally and physically
- Let go of the past and cut energetic cords
- Connect with your higher self and spirit guides
- Balance your energy and realign your chakras
- Manifest your desires and open to abundance
- Access peace, clarity, and divine wisdom

Stillness is your superpower. And your soul already knows how to find it.

The Resistance to Silence

If sitting still feels uncomfortable — good. That means you're on the right path. The ego resists silence because in silence, it has nowhere to hide. The inner critic, the old stories, the guilt, the trauma — it all starts to rise. And that's the point. Meditation is not about running from these parts of you, it's about witnessing them, forgiving them, and setting them free.

The thoughts may come, and that's okay. You don't have to fight them. Let them pass like clouds. You're not here to control your thoughts, you're here to detach from them. You are the observer. The witness. The awareness.

You don't have to be perfect. You just have to be present.

The First Step

If this is your first time meditating or truly turning inward, start small. Start gentle. This isn't a race to enlightenment. This is a journey to remembering.

Find a quiet space. Close your eyes. Breathe in deeply. Hold. Exhale slowly.

Do it again.

Let the world fall away. Let your body relax. Let your mind slow down.

Focus on the breath. Feel your chest rise and fall. If your thoughts wander, bring them back. If emotions rise, let them.

Allow.

Be.

Repeat a simple affirmation if it helps:

"I am safe. I am present. I am open to peace."

In that moment of stillness, you may feel nothing. You may feel everything. Either is perfect. What matters is that you showed up.

This is the call to stillness. And you have answered.

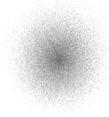

CHAPTER 2:

The Energy Body

You are not just flesh and bone. You are energy. Light. Vibration. The body you walk in is only one layer of your being. Beneath the skin, beneath the heartbeat, lies your true nature — an energetic presence that flows through and around you at all times.

This is your energy body. And when you become aware of it, you begin to take true control of your life.

The energy body is made up of chakras, meridians, the aura, and your connection to source energy. Most people walk through life unaware of this inner system. But once you tap into it, everything starts to shift. Healing becomes easier. Manifestation becomes quicker. Life begins to flow.

The Chakras: Your Inner Universe

There are seven main energy centres in the body, known as the chakras. Each one governs a different aspect of your physical, emotional, and spiritual self. Think of them as spinning wheels of energy. When they're balanced, you feel aligned, peaceful, healthy, connected. When they're blocked, you feel stuck, unwell, or emotionally drained.

Let's take a journey through the chakras:

1. Root Chakra (Muladhara)

- Located at: base of the spine
- Colour: red
- Element: earth
- Purpose: safety, stability, survival

When your root is balanced, you feel grounded and secure. You trust life. When it's blocked, you may feel anxious, disconnected, or fearful.

Affirmation: *I am grounded. I am safe. I belong here.*

2. Sacral Chakra (Svadhisthana)

- Located at: lower abdomen, just below the navel
- Colour: orange
- Element: water
- Purpose: creativity, pleasure, emotional flow

This chakra governs your joy, sensuality, and creativity. When open, you feel passionate and inspired. When blocked, you may feel emotionally numb or creatively stuck.

Affirmation: *I flow with ease. I deserve pleasure and joy.*

3. Solar Plexus Chakra (Manipura)

- Located at: upper abdomen, stomach area
- Colour: yellow
- Element: fire
- Purpose: confidence, willpower, personal identity

Your personal power lives here. It's the seat of your motivation and drive. A blocked solar plexus may lead to self-doubt, procrastination, or people-pleasing.

Affirmation: *I am strong. I am confident. I stand in my power.*

4. Heart Chakra (Anahata)

- Located at: centre of the chest
- Colour: green or pink
- Element: air
- Purpose: love, compassion, connection

When this chakra is open, you radiate unconditional love. You forgive, you empathise. A closed heart chakra holds onto resentment and fear of vulnerability.

Affirmation: *I am love. I give and receive love freely.*

5. Throat Chakra (Vishuddha)

- Located at: throat
- Colour: blue
- Element: sound
- Purpose: communication, truth, self-expression

This is your voice — your truth. When balanced, you speak with clarity and honesty. When blocked, you may feel unheard, timid, or misunderstood.

Affirmation: *I speak my truth with clarity and grace.*

6. Third Eye Chakra (Ajna)

- Located at: between the eyebrows
- Colour: indigo
- Element: light
- Purpose: intuition, insight, imagination

Your intuition and inner wisdom live here. This chakra opens the door to spiritual vision and guidance. When blocked, you feel disconnected or indecisive.

Affirmation: *I trust my inner guidance. I see clearly.*

7. Crown Chakra (Sahasrara)

- Located at: top of the head
- Colour: violet or white
- Element: thought / Divine Consciousness

- Purpose: connection to Source, enlightenment

This is your portal to the divine. It's your connection to something greater. When open, you feel at peace with the universe. When closed, you may feel spiritually lost or isolated.

Affirmation: *I am connected to Source. I am divine.*

Bringing Your Chakras Into Alignment

Each chakra is like a tuning fork. When one is off, it affects the harmony of the whole system. Bringing them into balance brings the body, mind, and soul into a state of flow — that beautiful rhythm of life where things unfold naturally, effortlessly.

You don't need to be a master to align your chakras. You just need awareness and intention.

Here are simple ways to begin:

- **Meditation:** focus on each chakra during your practice. Visualise the colour associated with each one spinning and glowing.
- **Sound Healing:** certain frequencies can activate and balance chakras.
- **Movement:** yoga, dance, and even walking can unblock stagnant energy.
- **Crystals & Oils:** use natural tools that resonate with each chakra.

- **Breathwork:** conscious breathing helps move energy through the body.

Remember: your chakras respond to your thoughts, emotions, and environment. Positive energy nurtures them. Toxic energy blocks them. The more mindful you are, the more aligned you become.

When You Align, You Attract

When your chakras are balanced, your energy becomes magnetic. You radiate peace, confidence, and love. People feel it.

You are now walking in high vibration. Opportunities begin to appear. Synchronicities guide your path. Life feels different — because *you* are different.

This is the power of energy. And it has always been within you.

CHAPTER 3:

Raising Your Frequency

Everything is energy.

Every word, every thought, every emotion — you feel it, carry it, and radiate it.

Your frequency is the vibration you emit. It's the energy you walk with, the unseen force that speaks before your mouth does. It influences the experiences you attract, the relationships you build, and the quality of your life.

When you raise your frequency, you change your reality.

Understanding Vibration

Think of your frequency like a radio station. You can't hear 98.5 FM if you're tuned into 91.3. The same goes for your energy. If you're tuned into fear, anger, or lack, you can't receive the guidance, love, or abundance that exist on a higher vibration.

Raising your vibration isn't about pretending to be happy or bypassing your pain. It's about choosing to be aware. Choosing to heal, to grow, and to shift toward what feels light, free, and true.

Your vibration changes when your perspective changes. And when your frequency rises, you begin to live in a new dimension of experience. You attract more peace, more grace, more alignment. Life begins to respond to your energy.

The Emotional Scale of Frequency

Each emotion holds a vibrational signature.

Here's how they generally align from lowest to highest:

- Shame
- Guilt
- Grief
- Fear
- Anger
- Frustration
- Doubt
- Neutrality
- Willingness
- Acceptance
- Love

- Joy
- Gratitude
- Peace
- Enlightenment

When you're feeling low — depressed, anxious, hopeless — it doesn't mean you've failed. It means your body and spirit are signalling you to shift.

The first step? Acknowledge where you are.

The next step? Choose something a little higher.

If you're in fear, shift to courage.

If you're angry, shift to understanding.

If you're grieving, shift to acceptance.

Little by little, you climb.

You rise.

What Lowers Your Vibration

Becoming aware of what drains your energy is key. Here are a few common blocks:

- Negative self-talk
- Toxic environments or people
- Holding onto the past
- Living in fear or scarcity
- Comparing yourself to others
- Neglecting your physical or energetic body

It's not about avoiding these experiences — it's about being conscious of how long you stay in them. What you dwell in, you become.

If something lowers your vibration, you can choose again. You can walk away. You can protect your peace.

What Raises Your Vibration

There are endless ways to raise your frequency. Here are a few that align with high-vibration living:

- **Meditation:** the foundation of inner stillness and clarity
- **Gratitude:** instantly shifts your focus from lack to abundance
- **Loving kindness:** giving love freely raises not only your energy, but others'
- **Movement:** dance, yoga, walking barefoot on the earth — move the energy
- **Laughter and joy:** lightness is medicine
- **Creativity:** singing, painting, writing — it's all divine expression
- **Being in nature:** the earth has her own frequency — let her align you
- **Acts of service:** giving from the heart amplifies the soul

Do what makes you feel alive. Do what makes your soul exhale. That's your frequency rising.

Faith Over Fear

One of the biggest vibrational shifts you can make is choosing faith over fear.

Where there is faith, there is no room for doubt. And where there is doubt, fear follows.

Faith says:

- Everything is happening for my highest good.
- I don't need to control — only to align.
- I trust the process. I trust the divine.

When you move from fear into faith, you create space for miracles. The universe rushes in when you make room for it.

Faith keeps you in flow. And flow is where magic lives.

Staying in High Vibration

This doesn't mean you won't ever feel low. You will. You're human. But your awareness gives you power.

The goal is not to stay in high vibration all the time — it's to return more easily.

Know what grounds you. Know what lifts you. Know how to reset.

Create rituals. Stay mindful of your habits. Protect your peace like it's sacred. Because it is.

You deserve to feel light. You deserve to feel whole. You deserve to walk in high vibration.

This is not just a lifestyle, it's a way of being. It's a return to your truest self.

CHAPTER 4:

The Subconscious Mind and Inner Dialogue

The most important conversation you will ever have is the one you have with yourself.

The words you speak internally — the ones no one hears but you — shape your reality. They create your self-image, influence your choices, and build the energetic field that surrounds your life. Most of this dialogue lives not in the conscious mind, but in the subconscious.

The subconscious mind is like the roots of a tree; hidden beneath the surface, but deeply responsible for how your life grows. It stores every memory, belief, trauma, emotion, and lesson you've ever absorbed. Some of these patterns you were taught. Some you picked up through experience. Some don't even belong to you — they were inherited from your parents, your environment, or even past lives.

But here's the beautiful truth:

- You can rewire it. You can rewrite it. You can reclaim it.
- Becoming the Witness
- The first step to healing the subconscious is to become the observer of your mind.

That voice in your head? It's not you. It's a collection of thoughts, fears, memories, and beliefs. Some are true, many are not. Most are old. When you start listening with awareness, you begin to recognise what doesn't belong anymore.

Ask yourself:

- Where did I learn this belief?
- Does it serve me or limit me?
- Who would I be without this thought?

That question alone — Who would I be without this thought? — can change your life.

Meditation helps you become the witness. Not to judge your thoughts, but to hold space for them, to gently question them, and to let go of what doesn't serve your highest self.

The Power of Inner Dialogue

Imagine if someone followed you around all day whispering things like:

"You're not good enough."
"You're never going to heal."
"No one really cares about you."
"You always mess it up."

That would be abusive, right? You wouldn't allow it.

But so many of us allow that exact voice to live inside our minds.

Your thoughts are energy. Every time you think or speak something — especially when repeated — it builds momentum. That's how limiting beliefs form. That's how identity forms. Your inner dialogue becomes your frequency.

Now imagine if that same voice said:

"You're doing your best."
"You are loved."
"You are healing, even if it's slow."
"You are powerful, and it's okay to rest."

What kind of life would grow from that soil?

You get to choose the voice you feed.

And when you change your inner dialogue, you change your entire world.

Healing Through Inner Work

To re-program the subconscious, you need more than just awareness. You need intention, repetition, and love. Here are powerful practices to help you go deeper:

1. Affirmations

These are declarations that create new beliefs. Speak them often. Write them down. Look in the mirror when you say them.

> *I am enough, just as I am.*
> *I am healing more every day.*
> *I am safe in my body.*
> *I am aligned with love, truth, and peace.*

Even if it doesn't feel true yet, say it anyway. The subconscious learns through repetition.

2. Journaling

Journaling lets you meet the self behind the thoughts. Try prompts like:

> What beliefs am I ready to let go of?
> What does my inner child need to hear from me?
> Where am I still seeking outside validation?

Write without judgment. Let it pour.

3. Inner Child Work

The most wounded part of your subconscious is often your inner child — the younger you who felt abandoned, unheard, unseen.

Speak to that child. Visualise them. Write them letters.

Say the words they needed to hear. Love them fiercely.

When you begin to re-parent yourself, you heal the foundation of your being.

4. Shadow Work

The shadow is not evil — it is the part of you that you've rejected or hidden away. It holds your pain, yes — but also your power.

To embrace your shadow is to reclaim the parts of you that have been lost to shame, fear, or judgment. When you integrate the shadow, you become whole.

Ask:

- What am I afraid to face about myself?
- Where am I projecting my pain onto others?
- What qualities do I judge in others that I also carry?

Don't be afraid of what comes up. You're not here to be perfect. You're here to be whole.

You Are Not Your Past

Just because you've thought a certain way for years doesn't mean you have to keep thinking that way. Just because something happened to you doesn't mean it has to live in you forever.

The subconscious holds the pain — but also the power. And now, with awareness, you get to choose a new story.

Speak life into your future.

Speak healing into your present.

Speak compassion into your past.

You are not broken. You are remembering. You are returning. You are rising.

This is the path of walking in high vibration.

And it begins with the way you speak to yourself.

CHAPTER 5:

Faith, Flow, and the Art of Letting Go

There is a current that runs through the universe.

It is invisible, yet powerful. Subtle, yet wise.

It knows where you are, and it knows where you're going.

This current is called flow. And to walk in flow is to walk in harmony with the universe.

But flow can't be forced.

It only reveals itself when you let go.

The Power of Letting Go

Letting go is not about giving up. It's not about weakness.

It's about trust.

It's about faith.

It's about recognising that you are not meant to carry everything, and you're not meant to control everything either.

Control comes from fear.

Letting go comes from love.

We hold on to so much:

- Old pain
- Past versions of ourselves
- People who were never meant to stay
- Expectations, disappointments, regrets
- The need to know *why*

But what if you didn't need the answer?

What if peace wasn't in understanding — what if it was in releasing?

Letting go is a spiritual skill. And the more you practice it, the lighter you become.

Living in Flow

When you are in flow, life doesn't feel like a struggle.

You begin to see divine timing at work. You stop chasing, and things start arriving. You feel guided instead of lost.

This is the space where miracles happen — not because you force them, but because you are aligned with them.

Flow is the natural state of a high-vibration soul.

Here's what flow looks like:

- You trust yourself and your path, even if you don't know the next step.
- You listen to your intuition more than your fear.
- You respond to life instead of reacting.
- You move with grace, not resistance.

The ego wants control. The soul wants connection. And when you choose soul over ego, you enter flow.

Faith is the Bridge

Faith is what carries you from fear to flow.

Faith says:

- I don't have to know how—it's not my job to know how.
- I trust the process.
- I believe that something bigger is holding me.

You don't need blind faith. You need heart faith; the kind that lives in your chest and whispers, "You are exactly where you need to be."

When you plant seeds, you don't dig them up the next day to see if they're growing.

You water them. You nourish them. You trust the unseen work.

This is what faith is.

And your dreams are growing, even when you can't see them yet.

Letting Go of Attachment

One of the greatest blocks to flow is attachment: to people, outcomes, identities, even desires.

Desire is not the problem. Attachment is.

Want what you want — but don't need it to be okay.

The paradox is: the more you let go, the more comes to you.

When you cling, you close your hands.

When you let go, your hands are open to receive.

Ask yourself:

- Where am I clinging?
- What am I afraid to release?
- What might be waiting for me if I let go?

Sometimes the very thing you're holding onto is the weight keeping you from rising.

Letting Go Is a Practice

This isn't something you master overnight. Letting go is a daily invitation. It may feel uncomfortable. It may feel like a loss at first. But with time, it becomes the most loving thing you can do — for yourself, and for your evolution.

Try this:

- At the end of the day, place your hand on your heart.
- Say, "I let go of what no longer serves me."
- Breathe.
- Feel the release, even if it's just a little.
- Let that be enough.

And when your mind tries to pull you back into overthinking, regret, or control, gently return to your breath. Return to your heart. Return to faith.

Trust the Unfolding

You are not behind.
>You are not lost.
>You are not too late.

Everything is happening exactly as it needs to.
>Even the pauses. Even the detours. Even the pain.

Life is not punishing you. It's preparing you.
>Preparing you to receive. Preparing you to rise.
>Preparing you to remember who you really are.

You don't have to carry it all.
>You don't have to force your healing.
>You don't have to figure it out right now.

Let go.

Breathe.

Flow.

This is how you walk in high vibration.

With peace. With faith. With trust in the unseen.

And the knowing that the universe is always working in your favour.

CHAPTER 6:

Trauma as a Teacher

No one walks through life untouched.

We all carry wounds. Some are fresh, some are deep. Some we speak about, others we bury. Trauma can shape our thoughts, affect our relationships, and linger in our bodies like a memory that won't fade.

But what if trauma wasn't just something that happened to you? What if it was something your soul chose to grow through?

What if your pain had purpose?

What if your wounds held wisdom?

This is the shift: seeing trauma not as a sentence, but as a teacher.

What Is Trauma?

Trauma is not just about what happened; it's about how your body and spirit responded.

It's the imprint left on your nervous system. It's the belief that gets formed in moments of deep hurt:

"I'm not safe."

"I'm not worthy."

"I'm not enough."

"I can't trust anyone."

It doesn't matter if the world tells you "it wasn't that bad" — if it hurt you, it shaped you. And your healing is valid.

Trauma can come from a single event or repeated experiences. It can be inherited through generations. It lives in the subconscious and in the body.

But here's the truth:

You are not broken.

You are healing.

You are remembering who you were before the pain.

The Purpose of Pain

The soul is not afraid of pain.

Pain brings awareness. Pain reveals what is unhealed. Pain breaks down the false identities and shows you who you truly are.

Your trauma may have:

- Taught you boundaries
- Led you to your spiritual path
- Opened your heart to others
- Awakened your empathy, your gifts, your truth

It may have cracked you open — but it also gave you depth. It gave you wisdom. It gave you *you*.

That doesn't mean you deserved it. It doesn't mean it was fair.

But it does mean you can choose to rise with it, instead of fall beneath it.

From Wounded to Wise

We have a choice: to stay in the pain, or to evolve through it.

To be the victim, or to become the healer.

To carry the wound, or to carry the lesson.

When you stop asking "Why did this happen to me?"

And start asking "What did this awaken in me?"

That's when transformation begins.

Your story may hold trauma — but it also holds triumph.

Healing Is a Journey

There's no deadline for healing. No finish line.

You don't need to be 'fully healed' to live, love, or walk in purpose.

Healing is not about forgetting what happened.

It's about releasing the emotional charge so it no longer controls you.

It's about choosing freedom, even when the past visits you.

Here are powerful tools to support your healing:

1. Meditation & Breathwork

Helps calm the nervous system and create safety in the body.

2. Therapy & Energy Healing

Modalities like EMDR, EFT tapping, reiki, or somatic healing help process trauma stored in the body.

3. Inner Child Work

Soothes the part of you that still feels afraid, abandoned, or unworthy.

4. Creative Expression

Writing, painting, music — all give your pain a place to be seen and transformed.

5. Community & Safe Connection

Healing doesn't always happen alone. You are not meant to do this by yourself. Connection heals.

Forgiveness: The Final Layer

When you're ready, healing often leads you to forgiveness.

Not for them, but for *you*.

So you can be free. So your heart can be light. So you don't have to carry their pain anymore.

Forgiveness says:

"I won't let this define me."

"I choose peace over bitterness."

"I honour my growth more than I hold onto my anger."

Sometimes, the hardest person to forgive is yourself.

For what you tolerated. For what you didn't know. For the ways you abandoned your own needs.

But you did the best you could with what you had at the time. And that version of you deserves compassion, not punishment.

Let Your Story Be Medicine

You don't need to erase your past to create a beautiful future.

You don't need to hide your wounds — they are part of your light.

Let your healing become someone else's hope.

Let your story be a bridge.

Let your voice be a torch for others in the dark.

You are not just a survivor.

You are a guide.
You are a healer.
You are rising.

This is what it means to walk in high vibration — not to avoid the darkness, but to carry the light through it.

CHAPTER 7:

Forgiveness and Detachment

To walk in high vibration is to walk lightly.

Not because your life has been perfect, but because you've learned how to release what no longer belongs to you. You've learned to set down the burdens that weren't yours to carry. You've learned to free yourself from the chains of anger, blame, and expectation.

This is the path of forgiveness and detachment — the art of freeing your soul from everything that weighs it down.

Forgiveness is a Gift You Give to Yourself

Let's be clear: forgiveness is not approval.

It's not saying what happened was okay.

It's not forgetting, excusing, or pretending.

Forgiveness is this:

I choose not to carry this pain anymore.

I choose peace over poison.

I choose freedom over control.

Forgiveness isn't about them. It's about you.

Your heart. Your healing. Your evolution.

We forgive to be free.

The Weight of Unforgiveness

Holding onto anger feels powerful but in truth, it drains you.

Resentment builds walls around the heart.

Bitterness keeps you rooted in the past.

It tightens your energy, blocks your flow, and lowers your vibration.

Unforgiveness says:

"You still have power over me."

"I'm still replaying the moment."

"I'm still giving energy to the wound."

You deserve to be free from that story.

You deserve peace.

How to Forgive

Forgiveness is not always one moment. Sometimes it's a practice. A decision you make again and again.

Here are a few soul-aligned ways to begin:

- Acknowledge your pain: Don't skip this step. Be honest with how it hurt. Feel it fully so you can release it fully.
- Speak or write it out: "I forgive you for…" — even if you never send it. Even if they're no longer here. It's about you.
- See the soul, not the story: Behind every hurtful action is someone in pain, someone asleep in their own suffering. Seeing the soul doesn't mean accepting the behaviour — but it helps you let go of the charge.
- Call back your power: Say it aloud. "I no longer give this person or this memory power over my peace."

And if you're still not ready? That's okay. Sometimes forgiveness starts with the willingness to forgive. The rest will follow.

Forgiving Yourself

Sometimes the hardest forgiveness is the one we owe ourselves.

For the times you ignored your intuition.
For the version of you who didn't know better.

For staying too long. For leaving too soon. For the mistakes you replay over and over.

Self-forgiveness is not weakness. It's maturity.

It says, "I choose to love myself, even through my flaws."

It says, "I deserve another chance."

You are not the worst thing you've done.

You are the light you choose to become.

The Freedom of Detachment

Where forgiveness frees the heart, detachment frees the soul.

Detachment doesn't mean not caring. It means caring without clinging. Loving without losing yourself. Moving through life with open hands.

To be detached is to say:

- I love you, but I don't need to control you.
- I desire this, but I'll be okay without it.
- I show up fully, but I let go of the outcome.

Detachment is a high-frequency state. It aligns you with trust, surrender, and flow. It opens you to receive from the universe without gripping so tightly to how it 'should' unfold.

What Can You Let Go Of?

Let go of needing to be right.

Let go of how others see you.

Let go of timelines and expectations.

Let go of relationships that no longer nourish your spirit.

Let go of identities that keep you small.

Ask yourself:

- What is no longer serving my peace?
- What am I holding onto out of fear?
- What would my life feel like if I released this right now?

Sometimes letting go is the highest form of love you can offer — to yourself, and to others.

Choose Freedom, Again and Again

You will be tested. You will be pulled back into old thoughts, old wounds, old attachments.

But every time you choose peace over pride, love over ego, release over revenge — you rise.

This is the path of the awakened.

This is the way of high vibration.

To love deeply, but hold loosely.

To forgive freely, but guard your peace.

To stay open, but never lose yourself.

Let go.

Let it flow.

Let yourself fly.

CHAPTER 8:

Relationships and Energy Exchange

You are energy. Everyone you meet is energy.

And every interaction — whether loving, draining, inspiring, or chaotic — is an energy exchange.

Relationships are more than conversations and chemistry. They're spiritual contracts. They reflect your vibration, reveal your wounds, and often serve as mirrors, showing you the parts of yourself that still need healing or are ready to shine.

Some people come into your life as blessings. Others come as lessons. Both are sacred.

But in learning to walk in high vibration, you must learn

how to manage your energy within relationships.

Not everyone is meant to walk with you forever. And not everyone deserves access to your frequency.

Understanding Energy Exchange

Every interaction has an effect. Some people uplift your spirit. Others seem to drain the life out of you.

This isn't judgment, it's awareness.

When you're around someone, ask yourself:

- Do I feel more alive, or more anxious?
- Do I feel expanded, or contracted?
- Am I being fully myself, or walking on eggshells?
- Does this person pour into me, or pull from me?

Energy doesn't lie. And your body knows before your mind does.

Protecting your energy is not selfish — it's spiritual hygiene.

Low Vibration Relationships

Low vibration energy shows up in many forms:
- Guilt-tripping
- Manipulation
- Constant criticism
- Emotional unavailability
- Victim mentality

- Envy, competition, or subtle control

You may feel drained, confused, or anxious around these people. Sometimes it's subtle. Sometimes it's deep.

And sometimes … you love them. Family, friends, even romantic partners can operate from this energy — often without even realizing it. This doesn't make them evil. It makes them unhealed.

But their unhealed energy isn't your responsibility.

Toxicity and Spiritual Protection

Toxic energy is real. It's heavy. It clings. It keeps you out of alignment.

Here's the truth: you don't need to fix them. You don't need to stay to prove your love.

Your peace matters more than their approval.

If a relationship consistently disturbs your nervous system, it's okay to:

- Set boundaries
- Say no
- Take space
- Leave if needed

Cord cutting isn't just symbolic — it's energetic.

You can release the emotional pull while still honouring the soul. You can forgive someone and still not allow them back into your life.

You are allowed to choose peace over history.

You are allowed to protect your light.

High Vibration Relationships

When you're in alignment, you attract relationships that reflect that vibration:

- Safe.
- Encouraging.
- Honest.
- Spiritually expansive.
- Rooted in love, not fear.
- Grounded in truth, not performance.

These relationships feel like coming home. You don't have to perform. You don't have to shrink. You can be real, raw, and radiant.

This kind of connection nourishes you on every level. You give, and you receive. There's harmony in the exchange.

High vibration relationships don't mean 'perfect' or 'conflict-free'.

They mean growth, safety, and mutual healing.

Relationships as Mirrors

Every person you attract is a reflection of something within you.

- The unavailable person might reflect where you've been unavailable to yourself.
- The over-giver may mirror your own need for approval.
- The soulmate who enters your life with ease may reflect the self-love you've finally activated.

No relationship is random. Every soul you meet is part of your journey — some to teach you boundaries, some to teach you love, and some to teach you what you'll never accept again.

Pay attention. Learn from each mirror. But don't live in someone else's reflection. Come back to your centre.

Maintaining Your Vibration Around Others

Even when you're surrounded by lower energy, you can still protect your vibration.

Ways to maintain your energy:

- Start your day with grounding meditation
- Imagine white light surrounding your aura
- Use affirmations like "I am protected and held"
- Limit time in draining spaces
- Practice emotional detachment from negativity
- Speak less, observe more
- Cleanse your energy (salt baths, sage, breathwork)

You don't have to react to every emotion or absorb every vibration. Not everything is yours to carry.

Loving Without Losing Yourself

To walk in high vibration doesn't mean you abandon love. It means you love wisely.

You can love people and still have boundaries.

You can support people and still say no.

You can offer light without dimming your own.

Love isn't sacrifice — it's synergy.

True connection empowers both souls.

So choose relationships that expand you. Let go of ones that deplete you.

Be open to love — but loyal to your peace.

Let Love Be Your Frequency

You are not here to fix everyone.

You are not here to stay small to keep the peace.

You are here to shine, to grow, and to attract those who do the same.

When your energy is clean, your connections become sacred.

You are love.

You are light.

You are worthy of relationships that feel like both.

Let your energy speak for you. Let your boundaries protect you. Let love be your guide—and your guide will never fail you.

CHAPTER 9:

The Law of Attraction Reimagined

The universe is always listening.

Not to your words, but to your energy.

Not to what you say you want, but to what you believe, feel, and expect to receive.

This is the essence of the Law of Attraction — not just a spiritual trend, but a divine truth. Like attracts like. Your outer world is a mirror of your inner world. And what you energetically emit becomes what you energetically attract.

But this law isn't about manipulating the universe with vision boards and affirmations. It's about aligning yourself so fully with your truth that you become a magnet for what already belongs to you.

To manifest from a high vibration is to remember who you are — and to resonate with what is already yours in spirit.

Manifestation Is Not About Getting — It's About Becoming

Most people approach manifestation from lack:

- "I want this because I don't have it."
- "I'll feel happy once I receive it."
- "I need it to feel complete."

But this frequency — this vibration of not having — is what the universe hears. And so it matches that.

The secret is not to chase what you want. The secret is to become the version of you who already has it.

When you feel whole, you attract wholeness.
When you feel abundant, you attract abundance.
When you feel love within, you attract love without.

You don't manifest what you want. You manifest who you are being.

Letting Go: The Paradox of Manifestation

The moment you need something to happen, you're pushing it away.

Need creates resistance.

Clinging creates fear.

Attachment creates blockages.

The universe flows when you do.

So how do you manifest what you want?

- Get clear on your desire
- Feel the joy of it as if it's already done
- Release the outcome
- Trust the process
- Act in alignment with what you've asked for
- Let it go

Want it. Love it. Align with it. Then release it.

That's the paradox: what you truly let go of, comes to you.

Manifesting from Service, Not Scarcity

When you ask, "Universe, give me more", you may unknowingly be saying, "I don't have enough."

But when you ask, "How can I serve?", you shift the frequency.

You build good credit with the universe through love, generosity, and contribution. When you align your desires with the greater good, manifestation becomes effortless.

Don't just ask for wealth — ask how you can help others

through abundance.

Don't just ask for love — ask how you can radiate love in every interaction.

Don't just ask for opportunities — ask how you can uplift and create meaning through your gifts.

The universe doesn't respond to begging. It responds to embodiment.

Emotional Frequency: The True Language of Manifestation

Your emotions are the signal you're sending out.

- Gratitude is magnetic.
- Joy is expansive.
- Love is powerful.
- Peace is receptive.

When you feel these states in your body — those chills, that open-hearted glow, that spark of excitement — you've entered the vortex of creation. You've aligned with Source.

This is the sweet spot where your manifestations take form — sometimes quickly, sometimes slowly, but always in divine timing.

Why Some Things Haven't Manifested (Yet)

Sometimes what you ask for is delayed because:

- You're still in a frequency of lack
- It's not in alignment with your higher path
- You're being prepared to receive something greater
- There's something to let go of first
- You've outgrown the version of you who asked for it

Manifestation is never punishment. It's always redirection, refinement, or divine protection.

Trust the delay. Sometimes the wait is the upgrade.

Daily Alignment Practices

To manifest from high vibration, make alignment your lifestyle. Here's how:

- Meditate daily to connect to Source and silence resistance
- Speak as if it's already true — affirm with belief
- Feel good on purpose — dance, laugh, walk in nature
- Act in faith — take aligned action, even small steps
- Express gratitude — before it arrives, as if it's already yours
- Serve others — give what you seek to receive

Let your entire being become a living prayer.

Let your life speak, not just your words.

You Are a Creator

You came here not just to survive, but to create.

To experience the fullness of life.
To dance with the energy of the universe.

You are powerful. You are worthy. You are magnetic.

The life you desire already exists in the energetic realm.
You're not trying to create it — you're tuning in to it.
You're remembering that you and the universe are not separate.

You are the vessel.
You are the vibration.
You are the manifestation.

Now feel it.
Now walk in it.
Now let it come to you with grace.

CHAPTER 10:

The State of Flow and Divine Timing

There is a rhythm to everything in this universe.

The tides rise and fall. The moon waxes and wanes. The seasons turn in their time.

Your life is no different.

When you understand the divine rhythm of the universe, you stop forcing, chasing, or stressing — and you start flowing.

This is the state of flow.

A place where your spirit, energy, and purpose align so fully that life begins to unfold with ease.

You don't hustle your way into flow. You surrender into it.

Flow is not about doing more — it's about being aligned.

What Is Flow?

Flow is a state where your thoughts, energy, actions, and emotions move in harmony with a greater intelligence. It's when:

- You feel present, clear, and grounded.
- Synchronicities show up without effort.
- Inspiration pours through you.
- The right people appear at the right time.
- Life feels guided rather than controlled.

In flow, you don't have to push. You receive.

You don't have to overthink. You listen.

You don't have to force outcomes. You trust the unfolding.

Flow is where the soul leads and the ego lets go.

The Conditions of Flow

To enter flow, your inner world must be aligned:

- Faith replaces fear
- Clarity replaces confusion
- Stillness replaces noise
- Presence replaces past or future fixation

Flow comes when you're not trying to get, but simply to be.

You enter flow by slowing down enough to hear your

own soul.

This doesn't mean doing nothing; it means doing only what's aligned.

Not every action is productive. Not every movement is meaningful.

Move only when your spirit says move. Speak only when truth rises in your throat. Decide only when your heart is clear.

Flow Is Found in Faith

You can't flow without faith.

Because flow will often take you into the unknown.

Your path may not look like anyone else's. You may be asked to release something you thought was 'meant to be'. You may be pulled in a direction that doesn't make sense, but feels deeply right.

Flow follows feeling, not logic.

Faith is how you walk when you can't yet see the road.

Ask yourself:

- Can I trust the process, even when it's unclear?
- Can I let go of control and follow what feels aligned?
- Can I believe in divine timing, even when it's not my timing?

The more you trust, the more the universe can move through you.

The Mystery of Divine Timing

Divine timing is not always comfortable.

It asks for patience. It tests your surrender.

It often works in silence — until suddenly, everything clicks.

Sometimes, things won't happen because:

- You're still becoming the person who can receive them.
- The path is being cleared behind the scenes.
- You're being guided to something better.
- You're being protected from something not meant for you.

The universe doesn't delay to hurt you — it delays to align you.

What's meant for you will not miss you. What's aligned for you won't require force.

Divine timing is a sacred trust fall.

And the fall always lands in grace.

When Flow Feels Far Away

There will be seasons where you don't feel in flow, and that's okay.

You are not failing. You are realigning.

If you feel off-track, return to the basics:

- Breathe deeply
- Sit in stillness

- Connect with nature
- Listen to your body
- Journal your truth
- Let go of what feels heavy
- Say no to what drains your spirit

Sometimes the fastest way forward is to pause. Sometimes the only way to hear is to be quiet. Flow isn't lost — it's just waiting for you to slow down enough to find it again.

Living in Alignment with Divine Flow

Living in flow means:

- You release attachment to the *how*
- You focus more on your being than your doing
- You live from the heart, not the habit
- You surrender to timing, not pressure

This doesn't mean life becomes perfect. It means life becomes divinely orchestrated.

When you're in flow, you're co-creating with the universe. Your part is to stay clear, stay faithful, and stay open. The universe handles the rest.

Flow Is Your Natural State

You were never meant to hustle your way through healing.

You were never meant to suffer your way into success.
You were always meant to walk in grace.

The state of flow is not a destination. It's a return.
　To peace.
　To presence.
　To Source.

So exhale.
　Trust the timing.
　Follow the pull.
　Let go of the struggle.
　And return to your natural rhythm.

This is the art of walking in high vibration.

CHAPTER 11:

Living a Soul-Led Life

There is a difference between a life that looks good and a life that feels good.

The soul is not impressed by titles, timelines, or trophies. It doesn't care how many followers you have or how much money is in your account.

The soul craves truth. Alignment. Purpose. Freedom. Expansion.

To live a soul-led life is to stop chasing what the world tells you to want, and start living from what your spirit truly needs.

It's not about perfection. It's about presence.

It's not about having it all. It's about being whole with what you have.

What Does It Mean to Live Soul-Led?

It means:

- You listen to your intuition more than outside noise.
- You make choices that honour your peace, even if they confuse others.
- You define success by how connected you feel, not how busy you are.
- You live in alignment with your truth, your values, and your divine path.

A soul-led life is not always the easiest path. But it is the truest path.

Let Go of the Old Blueprint

Most of us were handed a script:
- Go to school
- Get a job
- Find the partner
- Buy the house
- Stay safe
- Don't question too much
- Stay within the lines

But your soul came here for something deeper. Not just to exist but to evolve. Not just to survive, but to awaken.

Living soul-led often requires releasing:

- Expectations of others
- The need to explain yourself
- The pressure to be 'productive'
- The fear of disappointing those around you
- The illusion of control

You weren't born to follow someone else's path. You came to create your own.

Soul-Led Living Is Ritual, Not Routine

The soul thrives in ritual; sacred practices that anchor you to your truth.

You don't need a complex schedule or a 5 a.m. miracle morning to be aligned.

You just need intention.

Try weaving simple rituals into your day:

- A few minutes of silence before you touch your phone
- Speaking affirmations into your reflection
- Drinking water with gratitude
- Sitting in nature to ground your energy
- Journaling what your soul needs to hear
- Lighting a candle with a prayer of trust

Ritual isn't about control, it's about communion. It's how you return to yourself.

Integrity is the Soul's Compass

When you live from your soul, integrity becomes everything.

It's not about being perfect. It's about being real.

- You do what you say you'll do.
- You honour your boundaries.
- You speak with kindness, but also with truth.
- You don't abandon yourself to please others.
- You don't shrink to fit into old versions of yourself.

The soul has no interest in pretending.

It seeks freedom. Authenticity. Depth.

When you live in integrity, your energy becomes clear, and the universe reflects that clarity back to you.

Redefining Success

In a soul-led life, success is not defined by:

- How much you've accumulated
- How fast you move
- How many people approve of you

It is defined by:

- How deeply you've loved
- How true you are to yourself
- How often you choose peace over pride
- How fully you've honoured your purpose

Ask yourself:

- What would a successful day look like to my soul?
- What lights me up, even if no one is watching?
- What do I want to be remembered for?

Let those answers shape how you move through the world.

Let Your Life Be the Message

You don't have to be a healer, teacher, or leader to be soul-led.

You just have to live with love. With presence. With alignment.

Let your life be your message. Let your energy speak louder than your words. Let your joy, your peace, your wholeness become your offering to the world.

You don't need to know every step. You just need to stay connected.

Connected to your Source.

Connected to your spirit.

Connected to the truth that's already within you.

You Are the Masterpiece and the Artist

You are not just living your life — you are shaping it.

With every choice, every word, every intention, you create.

So create from love.

Create from truth.

Create from the fire in your soul and the stillness in your heart.

Live slowly enough to feel.

Live bravely enough to shift.

Live fully enough to know you honoured your soul, no matter what the world said.

This is the soul-led life.

Not loud. Not flashy.

But sacred. True. Unshakably yours.

CHAPTER 12:

Being the Light

You are here to shine.

Not because you've figured it all out. Not because you're perfect. Not because you're above others.

You are here to shine because you've walked through darkness and kept your heart open. Because you've chosen love, even when it was hard. Because you've done the inner work, and now your soul wants to radiate what it's found.

Being the light isn't about pretending you're always happy. It's about choosing to be present, compassionate, and aware in a world that often isn't.

Your light is your presence. Your energy. Your truth. Your kindness. Your frequency.

You don't have to force it. Just embody it.

Your Light Is Contagious

You may not even realise how many people you're inspiring just by showing up as your authentic self.

When you:

- Speak truth with kindness
- Hold space for someone in pain
- Walk away from drama
- Radiate peace in chaos
- Show compassion instead of judgment
- Choose healing over hurting

You are being the light.

You don't have to fix people. You don't have to convince them. You just have to live your truth. Your energy will do the rest.

Light doesn't preach — it simply shines.

Shining in a Dim World

There will be times when your light makes others uncomfortable. When people misunderstand your peace. When they resist your growth. When they project their own pain onto your presence.

Some may try to dim you. Some may question your path.

That's okay.

Not everyone is meant to understand your light. Some are still learning how to find their own.

Don't shrink to make others comfortable. Don't dim to make others feel less insecure. Don't carry the guilt of outgrowing what no longer resonates.

You're not here to fit in.

You're here to rise — and light the way as you do.

Light as a Form of Leadership

You don't need a title to be a leader.

Your light makes you one.

Whether you realise it or not, people are watching how you move through life. How you handle pain. How you love. How you rise. How you stay grounded.

When you live from integrity, truth, and compassion, you're leading.

Lead not with control, but with clarity.

Not with force, but with frequency.

Not by pushing others, but by being yourself so fully that others are reminded of who they are, too.

Protecting Your Light

Being the light doesn't mean letting your energy be drained by everyone who needs it.

You are not responsible for healing others. You are responsible for honouring your own energy so that you can show up with strength and love.

How to protect your light:

- Rest when your body calls for it
- Say no without guilt
- Cleanse your energy daily
- Spend time in solitude to reconnect
- Be selective about who gets access to your presence
- Set boundaries with love, not fear

Protecting your light is part of your spiritual practice.

Serving from Overflow, Not Sacrifice

You are not meant to pour from an empty cup.

You are meant to be so full of love, peace, and presence that it overflows naturally into your relationships, your work, and your world.

Serve not because you should, but because your soul is moved to.

Give not from obligation, but from joy.

Help not to rescue, but to remind others of their own power.

When you live in alignment, you don't have to chase purpose — it flows through you.

Let the Light Live in Your Everyday

You don't have to travel the world to make a difference.

Your light shows up in the small moments:

- The smile to a stranger
- The presence you offer a loved one
- The forgiveness you choose over resentment
- The integrity you walk in when no one is watching

Every time you choose love over fear, truth over comfort, stillness over noise, you're being the light.

The Ripple Effect

You may never fully see the impact of your light.
  But every high-vibration act creates ripples.

A kind word can shift someone's day.
  A compassionate presence can soften someone's heart.
  A soul in alignment can change a room, a relationship, a family, a community.

You don't need to be famous to be influential.
  Your light is already powerful, already enough.

You Are the Light

You've done the inner work.
>You've released. You've healed. You've aligned.

Now it's time to live your truth out loud.
>To walk in your peace.
>To serve from your joy.
>To speak from your soul.
>To radiate what you've become.

You are the light in someone's darkness.
>You are the calm in someone's storm.
>You are the reminder that love still exists in this world.

So shine.
>Shine without apology.
>Shine without waiting for permission.
>Shine because your soul came here to do exactly that.

CHAPTER 13:

Beyond the Body

You are not your body.

Yes, you walk in it. Yes, you care for it. Yes, you experience the world through it.

But you are more — so much more.

You are consciousness.

You are energy.

You are eternal light expressing itself in a human form for a sacred period of time.

This body is your vehicle, not your identity.

It is the temple, not the source.

You are not here to be the body.

You are here to embody your soul.

The Temporary Meets the Eternal

Everything in this physical world changes. It ages, it fades, it shifts.

But what does not change — what always is — is the spirit that animates you.

The *you* who watches your thoughts.

The *you* who feels deeply without always knowing why.

The *you* who senses truth beyond logic.

That is the real you.

That is the divine essence of who you are.

When you begin to live beyond the body, you start to tap into:

- The infinite wisdom of your soul
- The guidance of your spirit team
- The energy that connects you to all living things
- The universal flow that you are a part of, not apart from

You don't just see life — you begin to feel its sacredness in everything.

Awakening to Multidimensional Reality

This life is one layer of many.

Beyond the five senses is a spiritual reality that's just as real, if not more.

In meditation, dreams, or moments of stillness, you may have felt it:

- The presence of your guides
- The connection to ancestors
- The awareness of energy moving through your body
- The sense that you've lived before
- The clarity that comes without a single word

You're not imagining it. You're remembering it.

The soul is multidimensional. It exists in realms beyond the physical. And you, here and now, are simply a part of your soul's unfolding journey.

Life, Death, and the Sacred Return

Death is not the end. It is a return. A transition.

The body dissolves, but the soul expands.

After death, you shed the identities, the ego, the stories. You enter reflection, healing, remembrance. You reconnect with Source, your origin. You become part of the great light again.

And in that space, the soul reviews:

- What did I learn?
- How did I love?
- What did I come to evolve?

Then, when the time is right, the soul may return again. To grow. To heal. To serve. To remember more.

Life is a classroom. And love is the lesson.

Your Soul Has a Purpose

You did not come here by accident. You chose this life. This body. These experiences. This path.

Not to suffer, but to evolve.
Not to be perfect, but to become whole.
Not to escape the world, but to bring light into it.

Your soul has a mission. And that mission is always tied to remembrance.
Remember who you are.
Remember why you came.
Remember how powerful love is.

You are not here to fix everything. You are here to radiate your frequency and fulfil your piece of the divine puzzle.

And as you heal, awaken, and rise, you help others do the same.

Caring for the Vessel

Even though you are not your body, it is sacred. It is your home for this Chapter of your journey.

Honour it with:

- Nourishment, not punishment
- Movement, not stress
- Rest, not guilt
- Presence, not criticism
- Gratitude, not shame

Your body is the bridge between the physical and the spiritual. Treat it like the sacred vessel it is.

It speaks to you. Listen to it. It holds memory. Heal with it. It is sensitive to energy. Protect it.

When you love your body without attachment, you elevate your vibration.

Living From the Soul

To live beyond the body means to:

- See from your spirit, not your wounds
- Listen with your heart, not just your ears
- Move with purpose, not pressure
- Feel connected to all, not separated by ego
- Walk as if you are light — because you are

This is the awakened path. The high vibration way of being.

The soul-led life you came here to remember.

You're not just living this life — you're elevating it. You're not just walking through time — you're expanding through dimensions.

And when this Chapter ends, you will return to the Source.

Not as someone who was perfect, but as someone who was present.

Who healed. Who loved. Who awakened.

And that, beloved soul, is more than enough.

Final Reflection

You are not your name.

You are not your job.

You are not your mistakes.

You are not your pain.

You are not your past.

You are light.

You are love.

You are eternal.

You are free.

This body is your home — for now.

But your spirit is forever.

So live boldly.

Love deeply.

Forgive easily.

Shine brightly.

And never forget:

You are the soul. The light. The universe in motion.

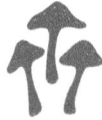

APPENDIX:

Daily Practices for Living in High Vibration

I. Daily Affirmations

Use these to align your energy with truth and intention.

Morning Activation

Repeat aloud or silently upon waking:

- I am grounded, present, and open to divine flow.
- I align with my highest self in all I do.
- I choose love over fear.
- I welcome synchronicity and grace into this day.

Evening Reflection

Use at night to release and restore:

- I let go of all that no longer serves me.

- I honour myself for showing up today.

- I am safe to rest, recharge, and receive.

- I surrender this day with gratitude and peace.

Chakra Affirmations

A daily scan using the 7 chakras:

CHAKRA	AFFIRMATION
Root	I am grounded. I am safe. I belong here.
Sacral	I flow with ease. I deserve pleasure and joy.
Solar Plexus	I am strong. I stand in my power.
Heart	I am love. I give and receive love freely.
Throat	I speak my truth with clarity and grace.
Third Eye	I trust my inner guidance. I see clearly.
Crown	I am connected to Source. I am divine.

II. Guided Meditation Scripts

These short meditations align with the themes of the book and can be adapted into audio or spoken practices.

1. Stillness Meditation (5 Minutes)

Use for centering, calming the nervous system, or resetting.

- Find a quiet space. Sit or lie down.
- Gently close your eyes.
- Breathe in through your nose... hold... exhale through your mouth.
- As thoughts arise, imagine them drifting away like leaves on a river.
- Repeat inwardly: *"I am here. I am now. I am peace."*
- Stay with the breath.
- Return gently to your body when ready.

2. Chakra Alignment Meditation (7–10 Minutes)

A visualization to balance and activate your energy body.

- Sit upright. Imagine a red light glowing at the base of your spine — warm, grounding.
- Move upward to an orange glow in your lower abdomen — fluid, creative.
- Then yellow in your solar plexus — powerful and radiant.
- A soft green or pink expands at your heart —

loving and compassionate.
- A bright blue swirls in your throat — your truth.
- Indigo pulses at your brow — your intuition.
- Finally, violet light opens at your crown — connecting you to Source.
- Breathe. Feel them spin in harmony. Say silently: *"I am aligned. I am whole. I am light."*

3. Letting Go & Surrender (For Anxiety or Overthinking)

Use this when you're clinging to an outcome or feeling blocked.

- Place one hand on your heart, the other on your belly.
- Inhale deeply… Exhale fully.
- Visualize what you're holding onto — an image, emotion, or thought.
- Picture it floating like a balloon into the sky.
- Say softly: *"I release control. I trust the flow. I surrender to the divine plan."*
- Stay with this release until you feel a sense of lightness.

4. Inner Child Healing Meditation

Use when emotions rise unexpectedly or when you feel wounded.

- Close your eyes and visualize your younger self —

any age that comes to mind.
- Imagine sitting with them, holding them.
- Ask gently: *"What do you need from me right now?"*
- Listen. Respond with love: *"You are safe now. You are seen. You are deeply loved."*
- Let the image fade, but keep the feeling of love close.
- Breathe deeply and thank yourself for showing up.

5. Flow & Divine Timing Meditation

For when you feel impatient, stuck, or unsure of your path.
- Sit in stillness. Breathe slowly.
- Visualize yourself floating down a peaceful river — you are supported, guided.
- Let the current carry you effortlessly.
- Say inwardly: *"I release resistance. I trust divine timing. What's meant for me flows to me."*
- Feel the peace of surrender.

III. Journalling Prompts for Spiritual Integration

Use these to deepen your awareness and activate healing.

Self-Inquiry

- What emotions am I ready to release today?

- Where am I being called to soften or surrender?
- What old belief still limits me, and what new truth am I choosing instead?

Subconscious Healing

- What did I learn about love as a child?
- Where am I still carrying someone else's energy or expectation?
- What does my inner child want me to remember?

Soul Alignment

- What does my soul truly desire — beyond fear or ego?
- What lights me up, even if no one applauds?
- Where am I being invited to grow right now?

IV. Rituals for Energy Reset and Alignment

1. Full Moon Release Ritual

- Write down what you're ready to let go of: patterns, people, pain.
- Light a candle or sit under moonlight.
- Read your list aloud. Then burn or safely tear it as you say: *"I release this with love. I call back my power. I am free."*

2. Daily Energy Cleanse (3 Minutes)

- Stand or sit quietly.
- Close your eyes.
- Visualize a waterfall of white or golden light washing over you from head to toe.
- Say: *"I clear all energy that is not mine. I return to wholeness."*
- Breathe deeply, anchor into your body.

3. Heart Opening Ritual

- Place both hands over your heart.
- Breathe deeply and smile gently — even if forced.
- Say: *"I soften. I open. I allow love to flow through me and to me."*

V. High-Vibration Living Toolkit

Quick Frequency Boosters:

- Step outside and connect with the Earth barefoot (earthing)
- Play uplifting music and move your body
- Practice 3 rounds of deep breathwork (inhale 4, hold 4, exhale 6)
- Speak gratitude out loud: 3 things, with emotion
- Drink water mindfully, with intention to cleanse and renew

www.ingramcontent.com/pod-product-compliance
Lightning Source LLC
Chambersburg PA
CBHW050034090426
42735CB00022B/3480